BOOK TITLE

INTERMITTENT FASTING: ADAVANTAGES
By Michael M. Walls

TABLE OF CONTENT

INTRODUCTION

What is intermittent fasting?

Intermittent fasting refers to an eating pattern that cycles between periods of fasting and eating. Your eating time is being scheduled in a way that you will be fasting and gorging on food. Historically, fasting has been practiced since ancient times. This is because, normally, at that time, people didn't have stores or supermarkets for goods, refrigerators to preserve food, or food available year-round. Hence, they were left to do fasting, even for a long period of time

Chapter 1

Turn on that fat-burning talent of yours

You know better than anyone that no magic pill will just sculpt you the perfect body that you want, but if burning body fat is your goal there are a few natural supplements that will accelerate the process. With proper training and a well-thought-out nutrition plan, Muscle and Fitness Hers will help you achieve your goals.

Starting a weight loss journey can be hard, and it's understandable to want results fast— especially if you're trying to tackle belly fat. Cue you, Googling, "how to lose belly fat in two weeks" to try to make this happen ASAP. Of course, weight loss is and should be a personal decision, and you should never feel pressured to lose weight. OK, but how do you lose belly fat? You have to think beyond crunches and planks and adopt a well-rounded approach. "It's got to be more losing fat routine Weight loss—and sustainable weight loss in particular—is usually a process that takes time, but there are some things you can do to speed up the process.

1. Accept that your behaviors will adjust.

1. A big part of weight loss is simply being aware of the decisions you're making. For example, when out at happy hour with friends, you may lose track of

how much you're eating or drinking. But if you take a split second to step back and become aware of that fact, you're able to course correct. "The awareness and then planning for what else I can be doing, that might give me the same benefit of eating comfort foods"

1. **Track your calories**.

2. The most basic approach to weight loss is burning more calories than you consume. For instance, since 3,500 calories equal one pound of fat, a weight loss app—or even just a pen and paper— can help you decide how many calories you need to cut from your diet or burn at the gym to meet your goals. "If you were to burn 500 more calories per day seven days a week, that would lead to 3,500 calories in a week and one pound of weight loss"

3. **Eat more fiber**.

4. Foods that are high in refined carbs and sugar don't tame your hunger, so you end up reaching for more.

Instead, eat more fibrous foods like whole grain bread, oats, vegetables, fruits, beans, legumes, and chia seeds. "They fill you up more," as fiber helps slow your digestion.

5. Women should aim for at least 25 grams of fiber per day (based on a 2,000-calorie) diet, according to the most recent U.S. Dietary Guidelines. Start with our high-fiber diet plan.

6. **Walk every day.**

7. If you don't have an established exercise routine, "walking is a pretty good entry point for people," Obese women who did a walking program for 50 to 70 minutes three days per week for 12 weeks significantly slashed their visceral fat compared to a sedentary control group.

8. "Even if your starting point is a one-minute walk, if that's more than what you've been doing, there are health benefits to that," One of the biggest mistakes people make when trying to lose weight is that they try to do too much too soon and get burnt out.

"Starting slow and working your way up is better than overdoing it and giving up,". An easy way to approach it: Commit to going for a quick, 10-minute walk after dinner, and slowly increase the time as you become more comfortable with daily movement.

Chapter 2

The weight loss benefit of health program

Being overweight or obese may cause many health issues. Similarly, losing weight rapidly is going to cost you your mental and physical health. For example, obesity might lead to diseases such as hypertension and diabetes. Therefore, weight loss may be crucial for obese people.

People try various methods of losing weight. However, losing weight slowly and over some time is much healthier. It comes with fewer health risks than drastic weight loss. Severe weight loss can lead to some health complications. Additionally, it can be hard to maintain.

Losing or gaining a few kilos throughout the year is normal. However, you can achieve healthy weight loss only through diet and exercise. Therefore, if you start losing weight drastically without even trying, you should consult a doctor immediately

- **What is drastic and rapid weight loss?**

Losing more than half to one kilogram per week is rapid and drastic weight loss. It is very appealing but, unfortunately, it may put you at risk of developing many health problems. For example, you may experience muscle loss, gallstones, nutritional deficiencies, weak metabolism, etc.

People follow special diets called "crash diets" to lose weight quickly. It involves eating fewer than 800 calories per day. It can be pretty dangerous. A healthy adult need at least 12001300 calories per day. Our bodies require adequate energy to perform daily activities without feeling fatigued. We also need it to maintain a stable metabolism. Having only 800 calories does not provide the body with the required energy.

People think that following a calorie-deficient diet is more manageable than exercising and helps to reduce weight much more quickly. It can help you burn fat fast. However, the body starts to lose water and muscle mass in that case, leading to many complications, such as dehydration.

In addition, it may show an overall reduction in weight. That is because the body starts using glycogen to meet daily energy needs. Glycogen is the energy reserve for our body. When these stores get used up, the body uses up muscles.

As a result, there is more muscle loss than fat. It is also challenging to maintain fast weight loss and quickly slide back into the old lifestyle and eating habits. It can also lead to the development of eating disorders.

- **Can You Maintain Rapid Weight Loss?**

You can lose weight by various methods. But the real challenge is maintaining the lost weight and keeping it off. According to research, people who follow crash diets may regain half of the weight they've lost within a year. They also have higher chances of retrieving all the weight they have lost after 3-5 years.

- **7 Risks of Rapid Weight Loss**

Muscle Loss

Losing weight and losing fat are two very different things.
Losing weight may not always be the same as losing fat. Although following a very low-calorie diet

(VLCD) helps you lose weight fast, it can result in muscle and water loss.

According to research, following a very low-calorie diet can deplete body mass. Furthermore, following a VLCD comes with some risks like muscle loss.

Metabolic Changes

Your metabolic activity plays an essential role in weight loss. Your metabolism determines how many calories you burn each day. In addition, metabolism helps convert the food you consume into energy. Therefore, having a fast metabolism helps burn more calories, resulting in quick weight loss.

According to a study, losing weight by eating fewer calories may cause you to burn 23% fewer calories per day. That is because your body experiences a drop-in metabolic rate. It may result from a change in hormonal balance. Furthermore, a reduced metabolic rate will result in weight regain.

Nutrient Deficiencies

Usually, people trying to lose drastic weight tend to skip meals, which causes nutrient deficiencies. While on a low-calorie diet, consuming essential nutrients like folate, B12, and iron can be very hard.

A deficiency of essential nutrients causes fatigue, hair loss, anemia, weakened bones, and poor immune function. Therefore, you should add more unprocessed, raw foods to fulfill these deficiencies. You will also have to add supplements to your diet in severe conditions. However, do not start on supplements without a dietician's advice.

Gallstone Formation

Gallstones are stone-like formations that develop due to undissolved cholesterol in the gallbladder. They can cause severe pain and cramps in the abdomen. According to research, losing weight drastically and rapidly can be a leading cause of gallstone formation. The gallbladder aids in the digestion of fatty foods. When you are not eating enough food, these digestive juices form gallstones.

Dehydration

Rapid weight loss is usually a result of reducing water weight or water loss. According to research, following diets that help reduce weight rapidly can lead to severe dehydration. It will cause symptoms like;

1. Discomfort
2. Fatigue
3. Headaches
4. Constipation
5. It can also lead to severe conditions like kidney stones or impaired kidney function.

Electrolyte Imbalance

The human body continuously adapts to minor changes to operate smoothly. But any extreme change might disrupt the body's reaction to biological stress, majorly electrolyte balance.

Electrolytes play a significant role in running bodily functions. They help the muscles contract and relax and also regulate heartbeats. Sudden changes in the diet can affect mineral intake, disturbing the electrolytes. It may lead to cardiovascular irregularities and put other organs at risk. However, the heart is at significant risk. Therefore, an electrolyte imbalance due to drastic weight loss increases a heart attack risk.

Fatigue

Following a crash diet can help you lose weight pretty quickly. But the extreme calorie deficit makes it difficult for the body to function normally. It can cause severe fatigue. As a result, it may increase the risk of fainting under minimum stress. Other symptoms include;

1. Irritability
2. Feeling cold
3. Muscle cramps
4. Dizziness
5. Constipation

It might also force you to go back to the original diet. As a result, you will find it challenging to maintain the lost weight.

• Causes of Rapid Weight Loss

Some people lose weight intentionally for better health.

However, there can be many reasons for drastic weight loss.

Some of these factors will make you lose weight without trying. Some causes are:

Eating Disorders

Having an eating disorder can lead to drastic weight loss. Anorexia and Bulimia are two such eating disorders. People with these disorders obsess over the idea of having a model-like figure.

Therefore, they take extreme measures to lose weight. However, it may lead to complications like vomiting or passing stools after a meal. It leads to drastic weight loss, but it is unhealthy.

Disease Conditions

Underlying health conditions are also a cause of drastic weight loss. For example, tuberculosis, HIV infection, and kidney diseases cause sudden weight loss. Therefore, it is essential to get regular checkups. It is also vital to follow a healthy diet. Consult a doctor and follow the prescribed treatment if you have such conditions.

Metabolic Diseases

Having a disturbed metabolism also results in drastic weight loss. People with hyperthyroidism usually experience this. It is essential to consult a doctor in case of such issues. Also, follow the prescribed doses of medications. Changes in quantities can also cause weight loss.

Medications

Certain medicines for thyroid, chemotherapy, and amphetamines may result in weight loss. That is because they suppress your appetite or interfere with bodily functions. As a result, they make you lose weight rapidly.

Substance Abuse

Narcotic usage leads to loss of appetite and dehydration, resulting in weight loss. In addition, using drugs indicates having an unhealthy lifestyle. An unhealthy lifestyle may cause you to lose weight and have poor overall health.

Healthy Weight Loss

Losing weight at a slow pace is beneficial in the long run. To achieve rapid weight loss, people follow very low-calorie diets. But according to a study, very low-calorie diets may not be sustainable. However, you can achieve healthy weight loss by reducing calorie consumption gradually. But, of course, you should do it with the guidance of a dietician to prevent any harm to your health.

Studies suggest that building healthy eating habits can help you achieve gradual weight loss. It also helps maintain a healthy weight for a long time. Including more fruits and vegetables, and reducing the consumption of carbonated drinks, and alcoholic beverages can be some of the healthy habits you can adopt.

Tips for Healthy Weight Loss

Losing weight at a slow and steady pace is the healthier alternative. It has a higher success rate at managing weight. Here are a few tips that you can follow to achieve weight loss at a healthy pace.

Include More Protein

Having a high-protein diet can help boost your metabolism, which can help you lose weight. In addition, it helps keep you fuller for longer without losing any muscle mass.

According to research, having a high-protein diet can have tremendous long-term effects during weight loss. In addition, it may also help maintain fat-free mass.

Include More Fiber

Adding soluble fiber to your diet can help with weight loss. It helps you avoid food cravings and reduce excess cholesterol. Fiber also helps improve digestion and improves bowel movement.

Reduce Refined Carbohydrates

Sugar and starch products are just a form of carbohydrates. A low-carbohydrate diet is beneficial for healthy weight loss. However, it is vital not to restrict them completely. You should include the correct type of carbohydrates in your diet.

For example, complex carbohydrates aid in weight loss because they take longer to digest. You can get them through oats, wheat, and other whole grains. On the other hand, refined carbohydrates lead to unhealthy weight gain.

Eat Slowly

Chewing your food properly helps to break down the food much better. On the other hand, binge eating and eating too quickly can make you consume way too much food. Instead, eat slowly and use smaller plates. It will help you control your portion sizes.

Green Tea

Drinking green tea or oolong tea can help your body improve its metabolism. It is important to remember that this does not melt fat. However, it helps the body burn more calories. It does so by improving metabolism. In addition, it has antioxidant properties, which are beneficial for your overall health.

Get Enough Sleep

Having a disturbed sleep cycle can boost ghrelin, a hunger hormone. In addition, it also lowers leptin levels, the fullness hormone. So having poor sleep can lead to increased hunger, making it difficult to lose weight.

Exercise with Weights

Resistance training includes weight lifting. Lifting weights doesn't only have to be for bulking up. It is also beneficial in burning calories. In addition, it helps prevent muscle loss. Include some weight exercises in your daily routine. Take the help of a professional trainer for better guidance.

Include HIIT Workouts

HIIT is High-Intensity Interval Training that involves a short but intense circuit of exercises. It helps promote anaerobic activity in the body, leading to calorie burn.

HIIT usually involves doing a superset of 3-4 high-motion exercises for 30-40 seconds without any rest. However, beginners can take breaks in between initially.

Summary

Weight loss is a subject of great interest in this era, especially crucial for overweight people but the way you lose weight and the time taken matters.

People who are overweight or obese should lose weight to improve their health. It prevents several metabolic diseases like hypertension, diabetes, and many more. However, it is essential to lose weight at a steady rate.

Rapid weight loss has adverse health outcomes. Although you need to create a calorie deficit, you should do it with the help of a dietician. Self-planned diets may result in unhealthy weight loss.

In addition, including healthy foods and being physically active is the first step. Avoiding junk foods is the second. Therefore, make simple lifestyle and dietary changes to lose weight. You can consult expert dietitians for personalized diet plans.

Chapter 3

- **Fasting Warning signs**
- There are several potential positive effects of Intermittent Fasting, including weight loss, better appetite control, and lower insulin levels. The main issue is that none of those benefits have been heavily researched in any way. The research is also the scantest in humans (compared to, say, the research in mice). It's also unclear if the root cause of the purported benefits is intermittent fasting itself (e.g. how it affects your body, say, on a cellular level) or simply the calorie restriction. So it's kind of trial and error at this point to see whether an intermittent eating style works for you and your body.
On the other hand, there are a bunch of possible negative side effects with intermittent fasting.
As mentioned, the upsides of intermittent fasting are still very much in the research phase – but there are some promising findings there. However, there's also plenty of anecdotal evidence that intermittent fasting does come with some possible negative side effects, and you shouldn't start an intermittent fasting eating plan without hashing those things out with your doctor first.

Here are 10 red flags to watch out for. And if you notice any of these side effects, that means stop intermittent fasting and talk to your doctor or a nutritionist before proceeding.

1. Feeling hangry

We're not 100% certain that "hungriness" is a real word, but it's a real sensation. This is the feeling of grouchiness, grumpiness, or overall irritability that comes with not being able to eat when your body is telling you it's hungry.

As WH previously reported, teaching your body to go 16 hours without food takes some practice, and some people's bodies might not ever be happy eating within a restricted window.

In theory, if you're consuming enough protein later in the day or at night, you shouldn't be starving first thing in the morning. But if you are, that's a sign you need to make some dietary adjustments during your caloric intake period to avoid turning into a major crank, or it's a sign that you're just not flowing well with fasting. For some people (e.g., those who work out a ton), not eating for long periods may just not be ideal for them at all – and that's something worth considering. Don't force it.

2. Fatigue or brain fog

Ever found yourself yawning over and over mid-morning, only to realize you never got around to eating breakfast? Since not eating breakfast is typically how most people do intermittent fasting, realizing that you're excessively tired every day – or making dumb mistakes because you're wading through brain fog – is a tip-off that you're not eating the right foods during non-fasting hours or that fasting isn't fitting in with your lifestyle needs.

"Pay attention to what you're fueling your body with, you can eat what you want on Intermittent fasting, but you should still be fueling it with good food that will make you feel healthy and strong." And if you just feel way better eating breakfast most days, listen to your body.

3. Food obsessions

Being on any kind of restrictive diet can affect your relationship with food, while some people like the rigidity of intermittent fasting, others may find themselves focusing way too much on when they can eat and how many calories they're getting.

Spending an excessive amount of time thinking about the quality or quantity of your food every day can lead to a type of eating disorder called orthorexia. According to The

National Eating Disorders Association, having orthorexia means you focus so much on "correct" or "healthful" eating that it has a detrimental effect on your overall well-being.

That shouldn't be the goal of any diet, "You want to focus on forming a healthy, positive relationship with food."

Read more: Would it be a terrible idea to try intermittent fasting while breastfeeding?

4. Low blood sugar

If you're having persistent nausea, headaches, or dizziness during intermittent fasting, that's a red flag that indicates the diet may be throwing your blood sugar out of whack. As WH previously reported, diabetics should avoid any kind of fasting diet for this exact reason: Intermittent fasting can cause you to become hypoglycemic, a dangerous condition for anyone with insulin or thyroid problems.

5. Hair loss

Seriously? Yup, sudden weight loss or a lack of proper nutrients, especially protein, and B vitamins, can cause hair loss.

An important point: While intermittent fasting doesn't necessarily lead to a loss of nutrients, it tends to be harder to eat a well-rounded diet when you're cramming a whole day's worth of eating into a handful of hours. If you think more hair than usual is falling out in the shower every day, re-evaluate the nutrition content of your daily meals and speak with your doctor about whether intermittent fasting is a wise move for you.

6. Changes in your menstrual cycle

Here's another side effect of sudden weight loss (which can be a result of intermittent fasting): Women who lose a dramatic amount of weight or are consistently not getting enough calories every day might find their menstrual cycles slow down or even stop completely. Women who have excessively low body weight are prone to a condition called amenorrhea, or the absence of menstruation. Sudden weight loss or being underweight can disrupt your typical hormone cycle and cause missed periods; so while you might be rejoicing in the way intermittent fasting has helped you shed pounds, you could also be depriving your body of the calories it needs to function.

If you stop getting your period and think it's linked to the intermittent fasting habits you're practicing, stop fasting and speak with your gynecologist to troubleshoot.

7. Constipation

All backed up? intermittent fasting could be to blame. "Any diet can cause an upset stomach if you're not getting enough fluid, vitamins, protein, or fiber," who emphasizes the importance of staying hydrated all day long.

It's easy, she explains, for people to forget to drink water during fasting hours – but going 16 hours a day without enough fluid is a recipe for (gastrointestinal) disaster. So if you've started an intermittent fasting diet and can't seem to get your bowel movements to happen regularly (or at all), it's time to hit pause on your plan and speak with a nutritionist or MD about what's happening (er, or not happening in this case!).

8. Unhealthy diet

Even if intermittent fasting doesn't trigger a serious disorder like orthorexia, it could still bring about some pretty unhealthy eating habits. In addition to not getting the proper nutrients, you could also find yourself making bad nutritious choices during non-fasting hours.

9. Sleep disturbances

Many people report improved sleep patterns while doing Intermittent fasting possible due to the way Intermittent fasting helps curb late-night snacking habits, and in turn, an inability to fall asleep because your stomach is busy still digesting that 10 p.m. nosh.

However, there is some research pointing to the opposite effect.
Diurnal intermittent fasting (meaning daytime fasting) causes a decrease in rapid-eye movement (REM) sleep. Getting enough REM sleep has been linked to all kinds of health benefits, including better memory, cognitive processing, and concentration, per the Harvard Business Review. It's unclear why exactly.

If you notice you can't fall asleep or stay asleep after you've started an intermittent fasting eating plan, again, hit pause and talk to a pro to make sure you're not hurting your health.

10. Mood changes

It would be weird if you didn't experience any moodiness or hungriness during intermittent fasting, at least in the beginning. And while some people feel a serious boost of energy or motivation once they adjust to fasting, it's important to remember that it is still a restrictive diet. Feeling obliged to follow it could have negative effects on your mood, especially if you're becoming isolated from friends or family members due to your diet restrictions.

If you're feeling down, anxious, or discouraged about IF, it's crucial to stop and get in touch with a registered dietitian, psychologist, or nutrition coach right away. They may be able to help you create a fasting schedule that better suits your mind and body.

Chapter 4

The End of calories

The intermittent fasting weight loss strategy involves setting periods where you avoid eating. Examples include the 5:2 diet, Eat Stop Eat, alternate-day fasting, and more. Many people find this simplified approach more helpful than counting calories.

There are many different ways to lose weight.

One strategy that has become popular in recent years is called intermittent fasting (1Trusted Source).

Intermittent fasting is an eating pattern that involves regular, short-term fasts — or periods of minimal or no food consumption.

Most people understand intermittent fasting as a weight loss intervention. Fasting for short periods helps people eat fewer calories, which may result in weight loss over time

The main reason that intermittent fasting works for weight loss is that it helps you eat fewer calories.

All of the different protocols involve skipping meals during the fasting periods.

Unless you compensate by eating much more during the eating periods, you'll be consuming fewer calories.

According to a 2014 review, intermittent fasting reduced body weight by 3–8% over 3–24 weeks (22).

When examining the rate of weight loss, intermittent fasting may produce weight loss at a rate of approximately 0.55 to 1.65 pounds (0.25–0.75 kg) per week (23).

People also experienced a 4–7% reduction in waist circumference, indicating that they lost belly fat.

These results indicate that intermittent fasting can be a useful weight loss tool.

That said, the benefits of intermittent fasting go way beyond weight loss.

It also has numerous benefits for metabolic health, and it may even help reduce the risk of cardiovascular disease

Although calorie counting is generally not required when doing intermittent fasting, the weight loss is mostly mediated by an overall reduction in calorie intake.

Studies comparing intermittent fasting and continuous calorie restriction show no difference in weight loss when calories are matched between groups.

Chapter 5

Quality of Food is important

So even though you are fasting, avoid high-fat, high-sugar foods, refined carbohydrates, and other poor food options. "Constant eating, even if you eat well, puts the body in a state of being signaled to 'build' which can be very taxing over time Pay close attention to the quality of the food that you are eating.

It's always best to select organic or locally sourced ingredients whenever possible to avoid any harmful preservatives or additives that can contribute to toxin build-up, or other health issues, in the body

The truth is intermittent fasting is much more sensitive to your eating pattern rather than the actual food you eat. Although, like any other diet plan and method, the goals are to lose weight, improve your wellness, and become healthier. Hence, eating a set of quality foods with your intermittent fasting is most effective for you. Eating these 9 foods while following an intermittent fasting method can surely help you hit your fitness goal.

1. Lean proteins

The feeling like your stomach is full can prevent you from consuming more food–and lean proteins can give you just that, most significantly, as you will be fasting for most of the time. With this full feeling, you will restrict yourself from eating.

Moreover, protein is essential to your overall health, regardless if you are on a diet or not. Proteins in your body help you build immune health and maintain muscle mass. Generally, muscle plays an important role in optimizing blood sugar balance and keeping your metabolism fast. Without enough proteins in your body can lead you to frailty, higher blood sugar and weight gain,

Some examples of lean proteins that you can eat during intermittent fasting are chicken breast, plain Greek yogurt, beans, tofu, and tempeh. Red meats are also part of proteins; however, eating a lot of fatty ones, like bacon and sausage, may put you at risk of cardiovascular diseases due to high fat and LDL cholesterol

2. Fish and other seafood

During your feeding time, eating fish and other seafood can be a great idea. Salmon and sardines are two of the most helpful to add to your diet as they are high in omega-3 fats and even protein, which can help in boosting health and reduce cellular inflammation. Some other kinds of fish and seafood you can consume are anchovies, crab, lobster, mackerel, mussels, oysters, rainbow trout, and shrimp.

3. Fruits with low sugar

Like any other dietary plan and method, fruits are essential in intermittent fasting. Fruits are jam-packed with vitamins, minerals, phytonutrients, and fiber, which are vital in sustaining your health while fasting. With the nutritional value of fruits, eating them can aid in lowering cholesterol levels, controlling blood sugar levels, and maintaining bowel health. Plus, fruits are generally delicious snacks with low calories; hence, you can eat them without guilt.

Nonetheless, a tricky thing with fruits is that they can be really sweet, loaded with fruit sugar called fructose. Overconsumption can give you metabolic health issues and may negatively impact your intermittent fasting results. Hence, better choose the ones that have low to medium amounts of sugar. Some fruits you can consume during your feeding time are apples, oranges, peaches, grapefruits, kiwi, pears, blackberries, strawberries, avocados, tomatoes, lemons, apricots, blueberries, and melons.

4. Vegetables

Of course, vegetables should be part of your diet plan. They serve as prebiotics in our digestive system, feeding your good gut bacteria for optimal function. Experts suggest that adding leafy greens to your diet decreases your risk of having heart disease, Type 2 diabetes, cancer, and cognitive decline. Some vegetables you should add to your meals are carrots, broccoli, cauliflower, green beans, kale, spinach, seaweed, cabbage, arugula, Brussels sprouts, celery, and asparagus.

5. Whole grains

Here's another nutrient beneficial for your intermittent fasting– whole grains, which offer a complete package of health benefits for your body.

There are three parts of whole grains, such as bran, germ, and endosperm. The brand provides B vitamins, copper, iron, zinc, magnesium, antioxidants, and phytochemicals. While the germ offers healthy fats, vitamin E, and B vitamins; and the endosperm gives carbohydrates, protein, and small amounts of some B vitamins and minerals. Overall, every part of whole grains is distinctively health beneficial.

Some whole grains you can consume are organic oatmeal, organic millet, organic quinoa, organic brown rice, organic black rice, and organic wild rice.

6. Beans and legumes

Eating beans and legumes in your feeding schedule is an excellent strategy while on intermittent fasting. These two are loaded with fiber, antioxidants, protein, B vitamins, and other vitamins and minerals that your body needs while it follows your new eating pattern.

Furthermore, beans and legumes can aid in balancing blood sugar, reducing LDL cholesterol, and promoting gut health. Plus, it keeps hunger and cravings at bay which is perfect during your fasting. Examples of beans and legumes are black beans, chickpeas (garbanzo beans), green beans, lima beans, kidney beans, and lentils.

7. Healthy fats

Generally, for people who aim to lose weight, fats can be a bad thing. However, healthy fats are essential for your body to function correctly. They are needed to support cellular health, energy, and hormone production. It also helps in insulation that keeps you warm and protects your organs.

Additionally, healthy fats should be added to your diet as they are necessary for metabolizing fat-soluble nutrients, including vitamin D, vitamin E, and multivitamins. In digesting herbs and spices like turmeric and rosemary, healthy fats should be present as well. These nutrients from vitamins need fat to be absorbed by your body.

Some sources of healthy fats are olive oil, avocado oil, coconut oil, MCT oil, ghee, avocados, nuts and nut butter, chia seeds, flaxseeds, and olives.

8. Herbs and spices

Herbs and spices provide a potent, powerful, and anti-inflammatory impact on your health. Yes, those that make your food more delicious are also needed in your diet, so don't cut them out entirely. Herbs and spices help in optimizing your intermittent fasting; hence, you must still add them to your meals.

These herbs and spices can be turmeric, ginger, cinnamon, cloves, sage, rosemary, and thyme.

9. Probiotics

Probiotic foods can be really helpful during your intermittent fasting. It generally helps you to have good digestion and metabolism. Experts suggest that probiotics balance the levels of useful gut bacteria and reduce irritable bowel syndrome (IBS). While on intermittent fasting, probiotics can improve your glucose tolerance, helping you to achieve weight loss.

- **Foods to avoid when on intermittent fasting**

Aside from eating quality, foods it is significant as well to avoid harmful ones. You must prevent yourself from eating foods that are calorie-dense and contain high amount of added sugar, saturated fat, and salt, including snack chips, pretzels, cookies, crackers, candies, cakes, and sugary cereals with little fiber, and granola. Also, avoid drinking fruit beverages and high sweetened coffee and tea.

- **Common methods of intermittent fasting**

The main concept of intermittent fasting is to have a time dependable eating pattern. Following this idea, several methods of intermittent fasting emerged based on the frequency and schedule of your eating. These are the following:

Alternate-day fasting – In this method, you should choose which days to eat or which not. Eating and food restriction is practiced each day alternately, whether you fast every Monday, Wednesday, and Friday, and the rest you will be eating with 25 percent of your daily calorie needs.

Whole-day fasting – this one is much more intense because you will have at least one to two days per week of complete fasting, while on the other days, you will have no food restriction, you can also choose not to completely fast the whole day but to eat only 25 percent of your daily calorie needs. One example of this is the 5:2 diet approach which practices a cycle of five days of no food restriction and two days of calorie restrictions to 400 to 50 calories per day.

Time-restricted feeding – this method of intermittent fasting is the most common one where you strictly follow a meal plan every day. Each day, there is a designated time frame for fasting and eating.

Chapter 6

Get your act together

Intermittent fasting turns on an important process called autophagy, in which your brain "takes out the trash" that builds up during the day. This self-cleaning process helps detoxify the brain, clear out old and damaged cells, and sweep away debris.

The most common fasting plans include:

16/8 fasting. This is the most common approach. It involves eating every day within an eight-hour window and then fasting for 16 hours after your last meal.

5:2 approach. This approach involves regularly eating five days a week. For the remaining two days, you limit yourself to a single 500–600 calorie meal.

Longer periods without food, such as 24-, 36-, 48-, and 72-hour fasting periods, may be dangerous. If you go too long without eating, it might encourage your body to store more fat in response to starvation. If you want to fast the right way, learn about the best methods and test them.

Benefits of Fasting

Mental function. When you fast, your body has less toxic materials flowing through the blood and lymphatic system, making it easier for you to think. While fasting, the energy you'd normally use to digest food is available to be used by the brain.

You likely won't notice this mental change until the first few days of a fast because your body takes time to adjust. You might have headaches or pain points at the beginning of the process. But after your body clears itself of toxins, your brain has access to a cleaner bloodstream, resulting in clearer thoughts, better memory, and increased sharpness of your other senses.

Healing rejuvenation. Fasting puts your body through a rejuvenation experience. It dissolves diseased cells, leaving only healthy tissue. There's also a noticeable redistribution of nutrients in the body. The body hangs onto precious vitamins and minerals while processing and getting rid of old tissue, toxins, or undesirable materials.

Increased willpower. Choosing to fast requires mental strength and the ability to resist short-term gratification to pursue long-term goals. When you choose to participate in such a challenging exercise and succeed, you'll likely experience enormous gratification and a renewed sense of accomplishment.

Tips to Use Fasting to Improve Your Well-Being

Ease into it. Try not to go from eating to not eating all at once. Instead, try to cut back on food and drink intake over a few days or weeks.

Avoid sugar. Food and cookies made from sugar can make you feel satisfied at first, but when your blood sugar goes down, you might become hungry and weak. To prepare for an experience like fasting, fill up on things like pasta, rice, meat, beans, and potatoes instead.

Cut back on activity. When you're fasting, try to take it easy on yourself. Try not to do much strenuous movement or exercise. Your body can't replenish itself when you're not eating.

Consider medication. Before you start a fast, check with your doctor about any medications you might take. If there are medications you have to take every day, talk with your doctor about whether it's OK to take them without food

Stop slowly. When you're getting ready to finish your fast, get back to eating slowly. Don't eat a huge meal right away. Instead, spread out your meals and let your body adjust and get used to the process of digesting food again.

Keep in mind that fasting too much or too often can be dangerous and cause dehydration, mental stress, and disrupted sleep.

Stop fasting if you:

- Have diabetes
- Have kidney disease
- Are recovery from surgery or illness
- Are breastfeeding
- Are underweight

Chapter 7

Structure of Fasting

Fasting is dependent on three types of energy metabolism: glycogen, lipid, and amino acid. As blood glucose levels fall during fasting, the pancreas secretes increased amounts of glucagon. This action also reduces insulin secretion, which in turn decreases glucose storage in the form of glycogen.

Fasting is a practice that involves a restriction of food or drinks intake for any period. Fasting has been practiced for a variety of reasons that range from dieting to religious beliefs to medical testing. It is commonly used in medical practice for blood glucose and lipid markers laboratory tests to aid in the diagnosis of numerous diseases as well as in assessing many risk factors. Variations of fasting have been studied for their ability to improve physiological indicators related to health. Some of these factors include insulin sensitivity, blood pressure, atherogenic lipids, body fat, and inflammation. Many of these studies involve those who participate in the Islamic tradition of Ramadan since participants abstain from food and drink each day from dawn until sunset for an entire month

The compiled results show a variety of metabolic and physiological adaptations that occur from fasting. From a general perspective, this includes the changes in metabolic pathways to create energy for the body

The effects of fasting have been thoroughly studied in populations of healthy adult individuals. However, data concerning underweight, geriatric, and pediatric patients is still lacking. A notable effect at the beginning periods of fasting is a tension-type headache. This type of headache has an etiology that is dependent on multiple factors and the precise cause has not been identified yet. Proposed mechanisms that might lead to a fasting headache include hypoglycemia, dehydration, along with caffeine withdrawal. A study has shown that the use of rofecoxib, a COX2 inhibitor, can be effective in reducing and even stopping a fasting headache, suggesting that the etiology may be a product of the pro-inflammatory eicosanoid metabolic pathway. Fasting should always be performed under the supervision of a physician or ideally in a clinical setting.

Cellular Level;

Fasting involves a radical change in cellular physiology and metabolism. Blood glucose normally provides the body with sufficient energy through glycolysis. During a fast, maintenance of blood glucose levels initially relies on glycogen stores in the liver and skeletal muscle. Glycogen is made up of chains of polymerized glucose monosaccharides that are used for energy by the process of glycogenolysis. Most glycogen is stored in the liver, which has the greatest role in the maintenance of blood glucose during the first 24 hours of a fast. After fasting for around 24 hours, glycogen stores are depleted causing the body to utilize energy stores from adipose tissue and protein stores. The drastic change in metabolism that follows glycogen depletion is primarily dependent on the metabolism of triglyceride stores in adipose tissue. Triglycerides are separated into free fatty acids and glycerol that the liver respectively converts into ketone bodies and glucose. Ketone bodies are made from free fatty acids through the process of ketogenesis. These ketone bodies travel through the body and are reconverted back into acetyl-CoA at the tissues requiring energy. In addition to adipose catabolism, protein catabolism, through the process of gluconeogenesis, simultaneously takes place in times of fasting. Gluconeogenesis produces glucose from amino acids broken down from various tissues including muscle. After glycogen stores become depleted, the dependence of body tissues for glucose gradually declines as ketone bodies become more readily available to metabolize.

Development;

One of the most heavily studied fasting regimens is known as intermittent fasting, which involves the restriction of caloric intake during a set period continually. Examples of fasting regimens include restriction of calories for 1 full day out of the week or 2 nonconsecutive days, also known as the "5:2" diet. Animal studies have repeatedly demonstrated a vigorous, positive response of various health indicators to intermittent fasting regimens. These include improved insulin sensitivity and a reduction of body fat, atherogenic lipids, blood pressure, and IGF-1. Animal models have also demonstrated a statistically significant improvement in the ability of intermittent fasting to delay the progression of neurological diseases including Alzheimer's, Parkinson's, and Huntington's disease. Human studies of intermittent fasting also demonstrate promising results in protection against metabolic syndrome and other lifestyle diseases including diabetes and cardiovascular disease. A notable cellular process that is upregulated during times of fasting includes the inhibition of the tyrosine kinase enzyme. Inhibition of this enzyme is a backbone for the treatment of many types of cancer, and further research is necessary to evaluate whether fasting regimens can be used concomitantly with chemotherapy to improve patient outcomes.

Organ Systems Involved;

The most immediate organ affected by a fast is the pancreas. During times of low plasma glucose, the pancreas will release more glucagon from the alpha cells found in the islets of Langerhans. Glucagon will mainly affect the liver as it stores most of the glycogen in the body. Skeletal muscle is also affected by glucagon, but to a lesser extent since skeletal muscle contains a low glycogen concentration. After hepatic glycogen stores are depleted, the body uses adipose tissue and protein for energy. The liver has an active role in the metabolism of fats as it is the main oxidizer of triglycerides. In more extreme versions of fasting, where fat sources have been expended, the body breaks down skeletal muscle for energy. Catabolism of skeletal muscle provides the body with amino acids that can be metabolized. However, this process also leads to a reduction in muscle mass.

Mechanism

Fasting is dependent on three types of energy metabolism: glycogen, lipid, and amino acid.

Glycogen;

As blood glucose levels fall during fasting, the pancreas secretes increased amounts of glucagon. This action also reduces insulin secretion, which in turn decreases glucose storage in the form of glycogen. Glucagon binds to glucagon receptors in the liver to trigger a cyclic AMP cascade that eventually activates glycogen phosphorylase. Glycogen phosphorylase and debranching enzyme release glucose-1-phosphate (G1P) from glycogen branches at the alpha-1,4 and alpha-1,6 positions, respectively. Then phosphoglucomutase converts G1P to glucose-6-phosphate (G6P). The final step of this process is that G6P is hydrolyzed into glucose and inorganic phosphate by glucose-6-phosphatase.

Lipid;

The breakdown of triglycerides begins with the activation of hormone-sensitive lipase (HSL). This enzyme is stimulated by glucagon, epinephrine, cortisol, and growth hormone all of which have increased plasma levels during fasting. Each of these hormones activates HSL through a different pathway. Glucagon and epinephrine bind to adenylyl cyclase (on the cell membrane) creating cyclic AMP. Cyclic AMP activates protein kinase A (PKA), which in turn activates HSL. Cortisol binds to glucocorticoid receptor alpha (GR-alpha) located in the cytosol of the cell. Activation of GR-alpha increases transcription of the protein angiopoietin-like 4 (Angptl4). This protein directly stimulates cyclic AMP-dependent PKA signaling which tells HSL to begin lipolysis. Growth hormone turns on HSL through the phospholipase C (PLC) pathway. PLC activates protein kinase C (PKC) which can either directly or indirectly stimulate HSL. The indirect pathway involves PKC phosphorylating MAPK/ERK kinase (MEK). MEK phosphorylates extracellular signal-related kinase (ERK) which directly phosphorylates HSL.

After HSL is activated, it works with adipose triglyceride lipase to break a fatty acid (FA) from triglyceride reducing it to a diglyceride. HSL and monoacylglycerol lipase break off the other two FA leaving a net total of one glycerol molecule plus three separate FA. Glycerol is converted to glycerol-3-phosphate and then to dihydroxyacetone (DHAP) by glycerol kinase and glycerol-3-phosphate dehydrogenase respectively. DHAP is then metabolized in the glycolysis pathway.

Fatty acids are transformed into fatty acyl CoA through fatty acyl CoA synthetase. Energy from fatty acyl CoA is mainly produced through beta-oxidation and ketogenesis. Omega oxidation is a minor pathway that oxidizes fatty acids into dicarboxylic acids in the smooth endoplasmic reticulum. It remains a minor pathway unless mitochondrial beta-oxidation is defective. The location of beta-oxidation is dependent on the length of the fatty acid chain; short, medium, and long chains are degraded in the mitochondria while very long and branched chains are degraded in peroxisomes. Every cycle of beta-oxidation produces 1 FADH, 1 NADH, and 1 acetyl CoA molecule. The very last cycle produces 2 acetyl CoA (from even-chained FA) or 1 acetyl CoA and 1 propionyl CoA (from odd-chained FA).

The process of ketogenesis first starts with the enzyme thiolate combining two molecules of acetyl-CoA into acetoacetyl-CoA. HMG-CoA synthase then adds another acetyl-CoA to create beta-hydroxy-beta-methylglutaryl-CoA. HMG-CoA lyase removes an acetyl-CoA group from the molecule to form acetoacetate. From this step, acetoacetate is broken down into acetone (by nonenzymatic decarboxylation) and beta hydroxybutyrate (by D beta hydroxybutyrate dehydrogenase).

Amino Acid;

During fed and fasting states, amino acids are generally used for the synthesis of physiologically important metabolites. Amino acids are metabolized based on their category and only the liver can degrade all amino acids. Glucogenic amino acids are made into Krebs cycle intermediates or pyruvate. Ketogenic amino acids are processed into acetoacetate or acetyl-CoA. There are amino acids that are categorized as being both glucogenic and ketogenic which means that they can be metabolized by either pathway.

Categorization of Amino Acids

Glucogenic: alanine, arginine, asparagine, aspartate, cysteine, glutamate, glutamine, glycine, proline, serine, histidine, methionine, valine

Ketogenic: leucine, lysine

Glucogenic/Ketogenic: isoleucine, phenylalanine, threonine, tryptophan, tyrosine

Related Testing;

Fasting is performed clinically when blood tests require minimal caloric intake to aid in the diagnosis of various diseases. Fasting blood glucose is an example of a test that helps to aid in the diagnosis of diabetes mellitus based on a set threshold that determines if a patient's insulin receptors are functioning properly by their ability to lower blood glucose in response to insulin. In cases of diabetes mellitus type 2, insulin resistance results in high fasting blood glucose. Additionally, high fasting blood glucose has been studied as a risk factor for the development of high blood pressure.

Another test that traditionally requires a patient to be fasting for accuracy includes triglyceride measurement on a lipid panel. Blood triglycerides are present in substantial quantity in the carrier proteins chylomicrons and very low-density lipoprotein
(VLDL). Chylomicrons are responsible for carrying triglycerides from digested food to peripheral tissues while VLDL is made in the liver and represents a baseline blood triglyceride level resilient to food intake. Therefore, an accurate measurement of blood triglycerides in VLDL requires a patient to be fasting to exclude chylomicron

triglycerides from the measurement. Recent data suggest that accurate lipid measurement may be possible in the absence of fasting although fasting for lipid panels is still recommended by most national and international guidelines.

Pathophysiology;

Chronic or excess exposure to glucocorticoids (GCs), such as cortisol, can lead to insulin resistance or even muscle atrophy. This type of exposure can be prevalent in more intense/prolonged versions of fasting. GCs normally relay their signal through the glucocorticoid receptor (GR) found intracellularly in skeletal muscle tissue. One primary action of GR is to regulate the transcription of target genes by either directly binding to DNA or tethering itself to other DNAbinding transcription factors. Inappropriate regulation of these target genes leads to the pathophysiological responses of GCs.

Clinical Significance

Fasting is not only important for clinically relevant tests but also has the potential to be used as a treatment for some diseases in humans. One study (sample size of 6) has shown that intermittent fasting, combined with the ketogenic diet, can be successfully implemented in pediatric patients with epilepsy. However, current literature on the subject is still limited and numerous studies still need to be performed to show the actual clinical efficacy of fasting as a treatment for human neurological disorders. Recent data also suggests that larger clinical trials are warranted to further investigate the efficacy of prescribed fasting regimens for the treatment of chronic lifestyle and obesity related diseases. Most studies related to fasting as a treatment for diseases have been based on animal models.

Chapter 8

Work out

Weight loss

Research suggests that during periods of fasting, glycogen stores are empty. This means the body starts to burn fat for energy during exercise, which may help weight loss. One study found that exercising in a fasted state also led to a higher fat loss than in people exercising after a meal.

Planning the workout

It is important to plan workouts during IF to stay safe. Some considerations are:

Type of exercise: There are two types of exercise, aerobic and anaerobic. Aerobic exercise, or 'cardio,' is exercise over a sustained period, such as running, walking, and cycling. Anaerobic is an exercise that requires maximum effort over a short period, such as weight lifting or sprinting.

Which type of exercise a person does will likely depend on the type of fast they do. For example, a person doing 16:8 or nightly fasts can do either aerobic or anaerobic exercise during their periods of eating.

However, if someone is doing alternate days and wants to exercise during their day of not eating, they should probably stick to less intense aerobic exercise.

Timing of the exercise: Although a person can exercise in a fasted state, it may be better to time exercise for after meals.

Type of food: If exercising during periods of eating, it is important to consider what to eat.

Pre-workout nutrition should consist of a meal 2–3 hours before exercise rather than just before. It can be rich in complex carbohydrates, such as whole grain cereal and protein.

A post-workout meal should consist of carbohydrates, high quality proteins, and fats to help recovery.

Safety Tips

After planning the workout, it is also worth considering the following tips to stay safe.

Exercising after periods of eating: This will provide a person with the energy they need to complete a workout

Sticking to low-intensity exercises: If in a fasted state, a person may wish to try and do low-intensity aerobic exercise. However, if exercising after eating, it is usually safe to do any type of exercise.

Listening to what the body is saying: If someone is starting to feel unwell during exercise while on IF, they should stop.

Staying hydrated: Even when not IF, it is essential to keep hydrated during exercise. As most of the human body is water, it is vital to replace fluids lost during exercise.

For some people fasting and exercising may be more dangerous, including:

people with diabetes people with low

blood pressure people who have

previously had disordered eating pregnant

women who are breastfeeding

CONCLUSION

In conclusion, our analysis revealed that Intermittent fasting was more beneficial in improving body weight, Waist circumference, and Fat mass without affecting lean mass compared to a nonintervention diet. Intermittent Fasting could also improve the condition of insulin resistance and blood lipid compared with non-intervention diets, but act similarly to Caloric restriction.

Different patterns of Intermittent fasting had different effects on metabolism. Moreover, the effects of Intermittent fasting were not uniform across women and men or in the overweight or obese population. More and larger multicentered studies are needed to evaluate Intermittent fasting while this study may lay a foundation for follow-up research to examine more extensively the reliable effects of Intermittent fasting.